This is for all those
hope, Because there is /

....

For my Mother and my son.

ACKNOWLEDGEMENTS

In memory of Jim Warner, who inspired me in our shared struggles with chronic pain, who always made me laugh in spite of it all. He'd have wanted to see this happen.

I would like to say a big "thank you" to Jason Pegler for turning my life around by agreeing to publish my first book. For his friendship, creative inspiration and positive attitude towards illness which has completely changed me as a person and given me my confidence back.

With thanks to Miguel Head for your confidence in my writing abilities. Many thanks to Tim Easun for his patience and help with the typing and scanning. I would also like to thank Kate Eliot for her inspiring support during the editing process.

To the chaplains at Nottingham Trent University for all their counselling and support during the writing process.

To Steve Ward, Jason Woolfe, Richard Morris and Simon Hinkerton for looking out for me during those times when the travelling made it more difficult to get about, and finally my classmates at Nosweat Journalism Training London, for being so understanding and accommodating as well as inspiring me to work hard.

ABOUT THE AUTHOR

This is a story by Fiona Whelpton, who suffers from a rare mental health condition known as 'Conversion Syndrome Disorder'. Causing heightened emotional responses, CSD makes the brain send faulty messages to the central nervous system resulting in limb paralysis. The symptoms are identical to Multiple Sclerosis. Fiona's case was so severe that she experienced episodes of interrupted walking, unconsciousness, and loss of speech.

Not knowing the diagnosis of her condition for four years led Fiona to try to find out as much as she could about what might be causing her symptoms. Switching on Radio 4 quite by chance she heard a discussion about psychosomatic illnesses describing her symptoms exactly, their subject was Conversion Syndrome Disorder. At last, after four years of tests proving negative (one of the main symptoms of the condition), Fiona was able get the correct medication and started to improve immediately.

In order to prepare for cognitive therapy treatment Fiona was asked to keep a record of her emotional experiences and try to link them to changes in her physical condition. Shocked by the scarcity of material on CSD Fiona realized that not only would writing help her recovery, publishing her story will give other sufferers hope and strength in the face of this rare condition. More widely Fiona hopes general readers will gain a unique insight into the experience of living with disability thus dispelling some of the myths and prejudices which surround it. Fiona is now planning to start work on writing a script for a stage musical based on The Cycle Path. She wants to promote a more positive image of disability by using disabled artists and actors, and accommodating disability into the choreography.

Now fully mobile, Fiona commutes to London from Nottingham twice a week to attend a postgraduate journalism course, and work experience with Jason Pegler at Chipmunka. In March 2004 Fiona was invited to a ceremony at the House of Commons, accompanied by Jason, where she was introduced to Lord Snowdon and received the coveted Snowdon Award. This £2000 bursary enabled Fiona to attend an NCTJ postgraduate journalism course at Nosweat Journalism Training in London, where she is currently studying for the NCTJ preliminary certificate in newspaper journalism. Fiona feels that her life experiences in Mental Health have equipped her to write feature articles about Mental Health issues. After the course she would like to travel to Europe to do some investigative journalism into the state of the Mental Health Services and treatment of psychiatric patients abroad.

Suffering from severe reactive depression for fourteen long years, then from Conversion Syndrome Disorder after the birth of her son, Fiona was hospitalized after a breakdown at 21 and some time later became pregnant during her time in a rehabilitation unit. This story is based on her life following the birth of her son. The names of the characters have been changed to protect their identities.

THE CYCLE PATH

This needs to be written down now, before it is too late to do anything about it. Having to cope with progressive disability means that one sees two sides to the coin. Somehow, one has a foot in both the "able-bodied" and the "disabled" world; seeing everything from both perspectives, but from different angles. The same as everyone else, and yet not the same.

The "able-bodied–disabled" person, whatever that means, is automatically excluded; is forced to be an outsider. People shut him out, ignore him, pretending that he doesn't exist. They see their own reflection in the mirror and wonder what life might be like for them if they were in his place. It might just be them, too. The "disabled" person watches their reactions from his wheelchair.

Somehow the barriers must come down. These fears and prejudices, based on sheer ignorance, prevent the "victim" from being everything that they have the potential to be. Passing the fear, from one to the other, prevents anyone from breaking free from fear and becoming a whole person.

CHAPTER ONE

I have decided to keep a diary, mainly to pass the time while I'm lying in bed all day here in the hospital. The days seem so long, there is nothing to do except just lie here. I'm strapped up to this piece of machinery which draws lines up and down; every time I feel as if I'm being kicked.

I have now been in here for three months, but it feels like a lot longer. There are so many people coming and going on the maternity ward, and I don't even know when I am going to have the baby yet. The nurses keep a constant eye on things. They say they need to get the blood pressure down, otherwise they think that I will have to have the baby by Caesarean section, not a pleasant prospect believe me. I think I am right in saying that it sounds a lot more frightening than a normal birth. At least you can hold the baby straight away. I don't think you can, after a Caesarean, especially not if you have to be put to sleep for it, which I have absolutely no intention of allowing them to do. I want to know about everything that is going on. The thing that worries me is that I won't bond with the baby, since I won't be able to put it to the breast immediately. I do SO want to be able to feed the baby myself. It sounds as if it is SO good for both of you. But they never tell me anything. Some people came in last night and have already gone home with their new baby, but I'm still here. WHEN is it going to happen? I am SO ted up of waiting ......waiting...... waiting......

I overheard them talking. They think I can't hear them, but of course, I can. They were talking about maybe inducing the baby if nothing happens soon. I wish it would. The nurses have come to see me again and informed me that it is necessary to deliver the baby immediately, and the safest way to do this is by Caesarean section. This has dashed all my dreams of a normal birth experience, and is not something that I feel comfortable with, but they have now given me the consent forms to sign and will operate in the morning. I will agree, but only on condition that they let me stay awake throughout the whole thing, I want Daniel, my partner to be there as well. At least that way, I might be able to see the baby immediately, I can't wait for tomorrow, I will finally see the baby.

*　　*　　*　　*　　*　　*　　*　　*

The birth happened a few days ago which is why I haven't been able to write any more up until now, because I wasn't feeling at all well. There is a big scar where they cut me open to get the baby out making me feel very sore no matter what position I tried to lie in and making breast feeding difficult, but everything went well in the end.

It was a little blonde-haired boy. Daniel decided to call him Matthew, after his brother. There was a worrying moment when the nurses were trying to locate Daniel, but they managed to contact his mother, who said that he was in the pub. Why didn't I think of that sooner? He was certain to be found there. He did manage to get here before they started the operation but was too drunk to be allowed in the delivery room. He was so drunk that he couldn't string more than two words together.

The doctors were concerned that they could hear an extra noise when they listened to Matthew's heart, but they didn't take him away for long, just to check him before putting him to the breast. He was very small, 5lbs – 2oz, with the loudest cry you ever heard. I can hear him screaming all over the hospital, and know instinctively when it's my baby crying, even when some of the others all start off at the same time.

I kept trying to feed the baby myself, but all Matthew wanted to do was fall asleep. In the end I had to admit defeat and give in to the pressure from the nurses to bottle-feed. I'd been so certain that breast-feeding was the best option for my new baby, but now it seemed that I couldn't even manage to do that properly. All my usual anxieties about myself started to rush back, much more acutely than normal. I really started condemning myself about my lack of confidence as a new mother, not realising that this was something most new mothers felt because of the hormones being all over the place during the pregnancy.

Something totally unexpected happened straight after the operation. When they put me back on the trolley to take me back to the ward I had absolutely no feeling in either of my legs. As I became more and more aware it seemed as if they were completely separate from the rest of my body. I grew more and more petrified. It was the most frightening thing that had ever happened to me. The doctor was very kind, and tried to explain that it was perfectly normal after an epidural.

*   *   *   *   *   *   *   *

It was three days since the operation and I still didn't have any sensation coming from the waist downwards. What would happen if I couldn't walk again, not ever? There'd be a small child running around and I wouldn't be able to move fast enough, if at all. I hadn't a clue how I was going to cope. The only thing I could do was to wait a couple more days to see if the movement returned, before making any major decisions about anything. I was so excited about having this baby, but the whole experience turned out to be a complete let down. It certainly wasn't anything like I was led to believe. I had hoped that becoming a mother would be one of the most special events in the whole world. But in reality it was nothing like it. Everything seemed to have gone wrong. On top of it all, the nurses were worried that Daniel was incapable of fulfilling his responsibilities as a father, and started expressing serious concern about his behaviour.

However, there were some things to be thankful for; the baby was really gorgeous, thriving in fact. The nurses suggested that we might be able to go home soon. The movement in my legs still hadn't come back in quite the way that it was expected to do, so the nurses decided to refer me to the physiotherapist.

The physiotherapist stuck needles all over me all morning and showed signs of being very concerned. Daniel might be able to help with some of the feeding now. They said I could possibly go home once things settled down with the legs a bit more. I hoped I'd be moving around more in a few days and couldn't wait to be able to get out of hospital and back in my own home again. All we could do was wait and see what happened. There was very little change in the situation with my legs.

*   *   *   *   *   *   *   *

The next morning I couldn't get out of the bed in the side room without help, and it took two nurses to help me walk to the ward and back. What would usually have taken five minutes took twenty. They decided that I needed to be kept in for at least another fortnight, which was probably just as well as it would give me and Matthew the chance to really get to know each other. How could Matthew possibly love somebody like me? I felt sorry for him, the poor child, having to have somebody like me to be his mother. Anyway, by the time that we eventually managed to get home, the midwife would be able to help sort things out, by which time I hoped to be feeling more confident. I knew I'd start to feel better if I were able to start walking again.

*   *   *   *   *   *   *   *

The nurses came to the conclusion that it was going to take quite a long time for me to be able to walk any better, and as Matthew was improving all the time, there was no reason why we shouldn't go home in the morning. They referred me to the physiotherapist for treatment from on a regular basis and at last, the day finally arrived when Matthew and I were free to go home. At least the house was cosy and comfortable due to a pre-admittance cleaning frenzy. Apparently it is perfectly normal to have very strong "nesting" urges when one is in the later stages of pregnancy.

I couldn't wait to get home and see the pets who were both delighted to see me. They always gave me such an enthusiastic welcome home and I really adored both of them. Ben, the sandy coloured, very gentle-natured Labrador and Bluebell, my grey and white cat. Labradors were supposed to be good with children. I didn't think he would mind about having a new baby in the house, I was more worried Bluebell might be a problem. I'd always been her "mum" and I thought she'd be quite jealous of the new arrival for a while.

I was still very worried about Daniel. Even though I was now at home, all he seemed to want to do was to disappear for hours on end to our local pub, "The Happy Return". He'd always tell me that he'd be in for supper and then cause a great scene if his tea wasn't on the table. We had a row about this one night. The baby had started screaming as soon as I had left him to start cooking and Daniel started complaining about the noise that the baby was making. He brought his fist down hard upon the table,

'Can't you do something to shut the f ----- brat up?'

'I'm getting the tea. Can't you see it's going to be ready in a minute?'

'Don't bother,' he snapped. 'I'm going out.'

I heard the door bang. His tea would have been on the table in five minutes but now I would have to leave it to keep warm in the oven. There was no way that I could go out and see him in the pub now that the baby was starting to settle down for the night. I had no idea what time Daniel would be back. I waited, and waited, and waited.

Quarter-to-midnight; it must have just gone closing time. Sure enough Daniel arrived back, but didn't come in to see me, he went into the lounge, chain-smoking, and turned on the stereo full-blast. It wouldn't be long before the sitting-room wallpaper, already yellowing with age, would be covered in brown nicotine stains and the room would stink to high heaven with smoke. I knew that the baby would wake up crying and it would take me simply ages to get him off again.

Another problem was Daniel's mother. She'd never really let her son go and he'd often spend whole weekends at his parents house, leaving me home alone with the baby. She would interfere to the extent of turning up at the house unannounced, bringing a single bed with her, then insisting that she put it in the lounge so she could make sure that Daniel got enough sleep with "the baby waking up in the night". Daniel didn't even bother to discuss my feelings on the matter.

I couldn't remember ever having a normal family weekend together. Daniel's mother always insisted that he go home for a "proper" Sunday lunch. It made me feel very angry when I thought of how many meals had been spoiled as he stayed in the pub for an extra pint.

The final straw came one day when my mother and I returned to the flat with the weekly shopping. Daniel had been drinking and had drunk himself unconscious. He was lying on the bed, the keys still in the lock on the other side of the door. There was no way of getting in so I had no choice but to take Matthew and all the shopping to my mother's for the night. Eventually we persuaded Daniel's father to go round to the flat. Apparently he had got very drunk and taken an overdose. An ambulance was sent for and after a stomach pump Daniel was put on a rehabilitation ward to "dry out", was the term I think they used.

*   *   *   *   *   *   *   *

Sometimes I just needed to be alone with my thoughts, all my friendships never seemed to go beyond the purely superficial level. At least

Matthew would fulfil some of those dreams. This is like being given a brand new start, having someone who is completely dependent on you.

At the moment I always seem to be anxious over every little thing, it's spoiling all the enjoyment of having Matthew at home.

My favourite times with Matthew were when I put him to sleep in the cot. I'd just sit there for hours, or what seemed like hours. These were times when I felt so close to him that the presence of any other adult would have been an intrusion.

My relationship with the baby was completely dependent on me and I was definitely not a good enough person to match up to that. I needed to make some sensible choices about Daniel, who was going from bad to worse. I absolutely dreaded payday. He'd go to the post office and then disappear all day, always returning drunk and usually in a nasty mood. All my dreams of having my own family were shattered.

It was such a relief that Matthew wasn't mobile. At least I could put him down, and know that he was in the same position as when I left him. But I knew this stage would pass only too quickly and that would be the start of all my problems. I still couldn't walk and Daniel was starting to frighten me. But I didn't really know what I was frightened of; him, the future, or the possibility that I might not walk again?

I was blissfully unaware that the operation had changed the course of my life forever.

CHAPTER TWO

Now Matthew is becoming more mobile, Daniel is much more of a danger to him than he was previously. He is so unaware of anything once he has been drinking, then he is sick everywhere, every morning. Matthew is always up so early, and all Daniel wants to do is sleep off his hangover. It is a massive shock to find out how physically active he is. I can't stop wondering what he is doing, not for a single moment. He's certain to have some disastrous accident happen, or make some big mess.

I remember the occasion when I found that he was able to get into the kitchen cupboard. There was a packet of chocolate biscuits in there. Matthew just opened the packet and began to munch one after the other until the packet was empty and chocolate was smeared all over his hands and face. He looked so guilty when I found him sitting on the kitchen floor.

'Matthew, what have you done?' I demanded.

He looked at me.

'It wasn't me, Mum.'

I really felt as if I was coming to my wits end. He wasn't old enough to start at the local nursery yet, although I thought his behaviour might improve considerably if he had the chance to play with other children more. I worried that he was lonely and frustrated by just having adult company. I wondered if I was projecting my own feelings of intense loneliness onto him, and that he was somehow picking up the atmosphere of this empty house.

The aching feeling of despair meant that I felt much too numb to be able to cry. I wanted to cry all the time, but there was a wall round me, stopping that from happening and all I felt was total numbness and emptiness. There were times when even the reliable comfort of Ben and Bluebell couldn't help me to escape the dreadful aching inside. Somehow this challenged me, made me want to fight these difficulties and turn them into something positive. Then it might help me discover the strength of my own character. I was very aware that I was at a crossroads in my life, and sensed that something deeply special and profound was about to happen to me.

The prospect of yet another evening without any adult contact or conversation makes me feel more empty and hopeless than ever.

CHAPTER THREE

When I woke up this morning I felt as if both of my legs had completely disappeared, as if there was no connection to anything below my waist. The only sensation I was aware of was a heaviness in both legs that I can't really describe as pain exactly, but was strange enough to make me feel panicky. I was conscious that although I still had some movement in both legs, I couldn't stand up without being in sheer agony. As I held on to the bed to prevent myself from falling I started to feel as if I had pins and needles in both feet as soon as they touched the ground. I asked Daniel to look after Matthew for ten minutes while I tried to have a bath. But when I managed to get downstairs Matthew and Daniel had gone.

I searched the whole house, high and low, but there was no sign of either of them. I felt panic overwhelm me; I wasn't walking well enough to go out looking for both of them. Half an hour later Daniel returned with Matthew and a can of beer in his hands,

'Why didn't you tell me you were going out? You should have told me.'

'Shut up you f -------- bitch. I'm going to my mother's.'

He slammed the door and disappeared. Matthew started to scream.

*   *   *   *   *   *   *   *

The last few days have been a complete nightmare. Daniel hasn't returned from his parents, and Matthew just keeps on screaming.

* * * * * * * *

Mum came round to help me with Matthew today. We were both getting him ready when he suddenly said,
'Daddy hurt me.'
My mother turned pale. There was deathly silence. I was sure she was in shock. Then she turned on me, 'You mean to tell me, that you LEFT Matthew ALONE with THAT man? I sometimes wonder at you.'
'I had no choice,' I protested. 'He seemed fine.'
'That's just my point, though. That you never know whether he's fine or not – and then it's too late… I am always so worried that he is going to hurt you or Matthew, or maybe both of you. You just don't know what he is capable of. How do you know what he might have done to Matthew – anything might have happened.'
How could I possibly live without knowing what happened? Maybe we would never know. In any case, it is probably better for all of us, especially Matthew, if we don't. Ignorance is bliss. But how can I forgive myself? I would have to live with the overwhelming guilt for the rest of my life and yet I still love Daniel. How can I love such a monster? Now I would have to make a choice between the two people I loved most in the world.

'I'm going to call the police,' Mum said. She moved towards the phone.

'That's not your choice to make', I said.

'What choice do you have, Fiona?' Mum asked. 'You are just going to have to choose between them. How will you ever be able to trust Daniel again, after this? Matthew is totally dependent on both of you. He comes first. He HAS to.'

The phone started to ring. I jumped. Daniel's father was on the other end.

'Where's Daniel?' I asked. 'I haven't seen him for a couple of days, and have been out of my mind with worry.'

'He's here – I'll pass him on to you.'

I waited, anxiously.

'Fiona – there's something I need to talk to you about', said Daniel. 'It's Matthew. I've hurt him, it's because I can't cope with the stress or any sort of responsibility any more. I've already been to the police and let them know. It's up to you if you want to press charges.'

'Charges for what?' There was silence at the other end.

'IT'S OVER. I'm leaving you.'

Feeling sick to the stomach, I sat down. My insides were churning, and as I asked Mum to call the health visitor, I found that my words were slurring, my speech was deteriorating. I was desperately struggling to make sense of all of this, and if I couldn't how on earth could Matthew? How could Matthew ever grow up being able to trust anyone after this?

The health visitor tried to reassure me that it wasn't my fault but I was still convinced this had happened because I was such a terrible person. Daniel was taken by the police for further questioning but apparently remained silent throughout. They couldn't press charges because they failed to say "anything you say may be taken down in evidence."

*   *   *   *   *   *   *   *

Evidence of what? That was something we'd never know, and still don't to this day.

A court case was arranged and happened a year later. I was granted a residency order, as they decided it was in Matthew's best interests to be allowed to stay with me. They took out an injunction to stop Daniel coming within thirty yards of us. If he did he'd be arrested immediately.

In spite of everything, I still loved him. I was entirely alone with Matthew and I had to begin again, alone. I was so afraid.

CHAPTER FOUR

As the sunlight streamed in through the bedroom window, I stirred, turned over and tried to get back to sleep, to shut out the too loud ringing of my alarm. It was six-thirty and if I didn't get up now Matthew would start screaming blue murder for his feed. I decided to put on my dressing–gown and head for the bathroom. After washing my face, I might start feeling more like a normal human being and able to face the day with a more positive attitude. But as I tried to move my legs I knew that this would be one of my really difficult days. I couldn't feel them.

There was no sensation coming from anywhere, waist downwards. In intense pain I eventually succeeded in managing to move my legs out of the bed and onto the floor. It took me ten minutes to get from the bedroom to the bathroom. But I knew that once I was able to find my pain relief, at least I would be able to start moving a bit further. I found it strange that sometimes I couldn't move for the entire day, and yet other times, if I struggled to get moving I could move better eventually. So it was imperative that I tried to keep moving and work through the agonising pain that was shooting all over my body.

When I finally got to the kitchen, both the dog and the cat were waiting for me behind the kitchen door. The cat mewed insistently, unable to understand that I had to put the kettle on. As I set about my usual chores both animals followed me around. I managed to ignore them. I would feel more civilized after a cup of tea. I knew that it wouldn't be too long before I'd be moving around again; the mobility seemed to return almost as quickly as it had disappeared. Some days it would be all day before being able to move properly, but on others I'd be beside myself with pain every time I moved. At least I COULD move. Something I'd come to learn that I couldn't ever take for granted.

I would have to phone my mother up for extra help with Matthew, this morning was evidently one of those days that would mean I would be out of action for the whole day. She would come over in the car and take Matthew off somewhere for the morning, for which I would be eternally grateful. Ben would just have to wait for his walk today. After lunch I'd take him down the flat cycle path at the back of the house. Letting him out for his run round the garden, I made a start on the washing up.

Sure enough, my mother arrived at the door to collect him. I could hardly manage to get to the door without having to hold to the rails to keep myself from falling over. I thought that I really should contact an occupational therapist to access the house to see if I could have it properly adapted, I couldn't carry on like this for much longer, that much was evident. Matthew was still upstairs refusing to come down when he was called. I found that I had to shout up to him which made me more wound up than ever.

I was absolutely determined I wasn't going to be beaten by the pain. I had to force myself to keep moving around; the movement would surely return if I kept going at all costs. The only way to do this would be to get out of the house and just walk to clear my head.

As soon as they had driven off I shut the front door behind me and gingerly managed my way up the path. I was in two minds whether to go and have coffee, or take a walk down the cycle path. I started up the hill to Sainsbury's but quickly changed my mind, realising that the cycle path would be the easiest option today.

Away from the traffic and noise of the main road the cycle path was pretty and peaceful, even though I knew I might find it busy with students cycling to the local hospital and university. I was getting slower all the time, the pain was spreading; I could feel it shooting through my entire body. Managing only a few more yards, movement left me; my legs went completely weak all over. I could feel their strength draining from beneath me. Feeling dizzier and dizzier, I passed out.

When I came round the only thing I knew was that I couldn't remember any more. Everything had gone totally blank. I felt as if I was surrounded by a big black cloud and had no way of working out where I was. All I could do was lie there, with my eyes shut.

The next thing I remembered was a voice that I didn't recognize, calling me. I tried to see who it was but found that my eyes wouldn't fully open. I sensed there was a tall young man, bending over me, but I had absolutely no idea who he was.

* * * * * * * *

Dear Fiona,

I hope you are starting to recover from some of the black-outs and that they have started to subside. Can you remember the first time I saw you? I remember it very well. It had been on the way to work, on the cycle path. I always choose that way, because it is so much quieter than walking up the bridge and along the main road, where it is so noisy at that time in the morning. I love the cycle path in the autumn in particular, there are so many different colours in the leaves as they turn russet, gold, brown and orange. The Pyranthia bushes along the cycle path look wonderful as I cycle past them on a crisp, frosty morning.

It was completely unexpected to find someone lying there. It is so unusual, especially to come across somebody unconscious as you had been that day. The strangest thing about the situation was that the paralysis kept coming and going, and I felt so sorry because you were obviously in a great deal of pain. My job as a doctor is to help people get better or at least cope with pain, but in your case I felt completely useless. My first responsibility, if I couldn't do anything for you personally, was to get you appropriate medical help. At least your house wasn't very far away from where you fell. You are incredibly brave, it must be so frightening not to be able to feel anything underfoot. My apologies for suggesting that you might be able to walk to the car. It was completely insensitive.

I hope that by now you are more comfortable, that you have started being able to move around a bit more.

Do let me know, without any hesitation, if there is anything I can do to help you. I will contact you soon.

Yours,
    Peter.

CHAPTER FIVE

When I looked at Peter as he offered to carry me to the house, it seemed as if he were connecting to my personality. He has a way of looking at you really closely, I love the way that a warm smile lights up the whole of his face. It's funny with some people, even though you've only just met they just don't feel like strangers. That's how it was with Peter. I felt completely at ease with him, even though it had been startling to find him bending over me when I wasn't too sure what had happened to make me fall unconscious. I'd never had a black-out before and couldn't remember anything either. But I felt so secure, and warm and safe when he lifted me in his arms. Somehow it felt wrong to ask him into the house but as soon as he had gone up the cycle path I deeply regretted not having asked him in.

Peter was so different from any other men that I knew; charming, very polite, caring and handsome. I had never seen such gentleness before, or such expressive eyes. Even though my vulnerability meant that I had no choice but to let him go, I was conscious of how desperately I wanted him to stay. He made sure I was safe and then had to leave, making me feel lonelier than ever. I had felt a sense of inevitability throughout the whole of that morning and now I found myself longing to hear from him again.

I felt much more content about everything than I normally do after having to deal with one of my episodes of paralysis. Usually I found it really hard having to be alone, and the extra burden of so much physical pain made it even harder to bear.

Whenever I become physically disabled, I find myself fighting a whole mixture of different emotions. I seem to spend a lot of time hating myself, because there are so many walls between me and anyone who is able-bodied. There is an immediate sense of isolation. Most people don't know how to approach me when I become ill, they stare at me coldly and walk straight past, not wanting to get involved. When I get home, I always seem to turn the blame in on myself. If I were like other people I would be able to make contact straight away, but there are so many problems caused by the simple fact that I just can't stand up to have a normal conversation for any length of time. I put up barriers of shyness. It prevents people who try to talk to me from becoming too close. I do this because I am frightened of being found out.

Sometimes the disability can almost be an advantage. To the outsider it is immediately a disadvantage, but for the person behind the disability, it can be used to its full advantage. One can "pretend" to be helpless. One can hide behind "the mask". There are very few people with whom I feel comfortable enough to show my real self; if they want to look beyond the mask that's up to them. When I fall over, people don't even bother to come and help, they are too embarrassed. That is why this morning had been so unusual, and why I hadn't been able to stop thinking about the young man.

Usually it takes a while before I can start moving around again properly, but today was different, I felt cheerful, almost hopeful about life. I think I was even starting to feel more positive. What was even stranger was that I didn't tell anybody, not Matthew or even my mother, about what happened that day.

*   *   *   *   *   *   *   *

Over the next few weeks we saw Peter several times. He knew just the right way to handle Matthew and always had a calming effect on me.

CHAPTER SIX

It was a gorgeous, warm and sunny July morning. Despite this, it turned out to be totally frustrating. I tried to offer Matthew a variety of activities, none of which he was willing to cooperate with. It was clear he was bored to tears; he could be so difficult and restless, climbing all over my furniture, turning the living room into a gym, using the sofa as a trampoline. Then he started on his usual demanding tactics, 'Why do we have to stay here?' he demanded. 'I want to go out, and find somewhere where there are other children to play with.'

It would be really nice to take Matthew out of the house for a while .There was a play scheme for children of all ages in Unity House, the community centre on Church Street, where he could play with other kids his own age. It would be good for him and I was starting to feel more and more stressed. I could feel my temper reaching boiling point, as I had to spend much of my time telling Matthew off. It wouldn't be long before it got out of control and I would end up smacking him, which I always felt I so ashamed of doing.

I thought it was one of my good days for I was at least walking. On the bad days, especially, I could have done with the chance to get Matthew out where there was more space to move around, and at least he would have other children to play with. I always seemed to have to stop him from climbing. It was at times like this that I felt really angry with my ex-partner, Daniel, for not being there, but knew it was better for Matthew and I to struggle on than to allow him anywhere near to help.

I felt that the holiday club was our only chance of survival, but now Matthew had started arguing with me, while I had been trying to put his coat on. How I managed to get him out of the front door, without smacking him, is beyond me. The best thing to do was to pretend that I was deaf, as Matthew had decided to start screaming while we both walked down the main road. When we turned the corner to go into Church Street he let go of my hand and tore off in the direction of the graveyard. I felt very worried and then my legs started to feel as if they were going from underneath me. Somehow I managed to get inside Unity House. Fortunately Peter was one of the students who had been assigned to welcome the parents in.

'What's wrong?' he asked me straight away. 'Is there anything I can do?'

The kindness on his face was almost too much to bear, and I burst into floods of tears. There were no more words spoken between us, there was no need. Peter went off to the graveyard, and ten minutes later, had found Matthew. He took him inside and asked someone to make me a sandwich and a cup of tea. He said that on no account was I to go home until I felt calmer. I suddenly felt as if someone understood.

'Would you like to stay and watch, while I help the children to make some bread?' Peter offered.

The children followed him into the kitchen, where bowls were set around the tabletop. They stood, two to a bowl, waiting eagerly for instructions. The flour was measured, water and yeast mixed to exactly the right temperature. Peter started trying to show the children how to knead the dough so that it stretched in precisely the right way, then he folded it over, and worked into it with his hands, each time the dough got bigger. I was observing him carefully, taking in every single feature – his tallness, fairness, and radiant blue eyes, but the most striking feature of all was the underlying masculinity, which seemed to come from his gentleness.

My emotions were completely uncontrollable every time I was near him. Joy surged right through me each time I looked into his eyes. I had to hide the fact that I was starting to have feelings towards him I didn't want. But I had no choice. I tried to shake the feelings off, tried to rationalize them, but even as I tried to make sense of the sudden outpouring of emotions, which were bubbling inside like a waterfall, nothing made sense. Anyway, why did it have to make sense? I knew that no one else had ever made me feel this way before and that there was absolutely nothing I could do about it.

As I watched Peter I told myself to stop being so ridiculous, I hardly knew anything about him. But he had just given me a real feeling of self-confidence; he made me feel as if I mattered. There was one question I had been burning to ask him, but even though I had it on the tip of my tongue I kept holding back. I wanted to ask the dreaded question: "How old are you?". As if it mattered. But he is so independent, has a car, a job, and a promising future ahead of him as a doctor. I knew that medical training takes a long time – years actually and I realised that I'd rather not know. Why? Was it because it was already too late, the young man had already made a tremendous impact on me. Maybe – 'If only ….' I sighed.

Life had been full of "if onlys." Peter smiled at me, and sheer joy welled up inside, overtaking all my insecurities and fears. 'What will be, will be,' I said to myself.

Matthew had been completely preoccupied with the bread making, and for once he was quiet. The young man's gentle character had rubbed off on him, too. Matthew had definitely become less jumpy. Having someone who would be able to run about with my son could only be a good thing.

I knew that mum would become extremely confrontational about the age issue, and probably add to the awkwardness by causing an embarrassing scene in front of Peter. But I was loath to confront the issues myself, for I had started to feel hopeful and positive about everything for the first time in a very long while. Especially with the prospect of regular help from him with Matthew, which would give me the chance to get to know him properly?

Peter ended up spending every free weekend with us, calling round to take Matthew out to the park, or both of us for long country walks. He felt that regular outings to the country would help me deal with my problems with stress as well as giving Matthew the chance of fresh air and exercise, as he'd be able to run around freely without me constantly having to worry about him.

CHAPTER SEVEN

One day Peter suggested to me that it might be a good idea if he were to come home with us and play ball with Matthew, so that he would be able to let off some of his energy. 'Come back for lunch,' I said. Then I found I was, again, unreasonably happy.

I found myself becoming automatically cautious, because if I allowed myself to be happy about anything in the past it had always turned out to have a detrimental effect on me, and everything I hoped for always ended up going wrong. So it was easier to go into denial. As I looked at Peter I suddenly realized that the feeling that there was always something missing had gone. Maybe this was what had been missing all along. I felt the air turn completely chilly. For a split second I felt desperately afraid, so frightened that I started to feel sick with fear. I tried to reason with my emotions. How could someone as kind as Peter seemed to be do anyone any harm?

I tried to brush my insecurities aside but it wasn't any use. I realized that the sense of foreboding was much more powerful than any of the other emotions, the longing, happiness, or joy that I had experienced in the short space of time that I had known Peter. Why was I so afraid? Was I afraid of the future?

Walking home with Peter and Matthew I realized that I had to choose to trust someone. All my life I had mistrusted anyone who had tried to get closer than the average friendship allowed room for. I realized that if I didn't take any risks now, then I'd spend the rest of my life feeling lonely. I had to take a positive step towards changing that situation. That meant I'd have to take risks, costly risks; it wasn't just my life that was being affected, but Matthew's as well.

I went to prepare lunch for the three of us and watched them kicking the ball together through the kitchen window. Matthew absolutely worshipped Peter already. If I didn't grab the chance of happiness now, and I'd be mad not to, I'd never be happy. Perhaps it would be safer never to be happy than to make a mistake. Why not just enjoy things and relax? Then I thought about my mother. There was a loud knock at the door.

'Aren't you going to let me in?' Mum asked. 'Where's Matthew?'

'Outside.'

She pushed past me into the kitchen, where the back door stood open. Ben was barking noisily.

'He's a very handsome fellow,' she said.

I ignored her, not wishing to give anything away.

'He's very blonde. He looks German, is he?'

'No, He comes from Cornwall, actually, he's a medical student.'

'He looks so young, he's only a boy. Do you know how old he is?'

'I don't know,' I said truthfully.

'Then if you won't ask him, I'm going to. If he's going to spend any amount of time with my grandson, then things like that are important.

Hasn't he got the most expressive eyes, though?' she commented, making me blush bright red with embarrassment.

I was thankful that Peter was kicking the ball around outside. He was blissfully unaware of my Mother's antagonistic attitude towards him. She was always extremely over-protective as soon as anyone new came anywhere near me or Matthew.

'I have another question,' said my mother. 'How come somebody who is as attractive as he is, is still single at his age? I would have thought most people would have found him impossible to resist, not with looks like that.'

'As far as I know, he has never had a girlfriend'

'What??!!!' she went extremely pale. 'Do you think there is any possibility that he may be gay?

'Oh, for goodness sake mother,' I snapped, now highly irritated by my mother's scrutiny.

Mum could always be guaranteed to come out with extremely narrow-minded comments.

'He's a medical student. Have you any idea how long junior doctors are working, nowadays? They work all the hours God sends. Peter is on so many nightshifts that he has absolutely no time left to develop any kind of social life at all.'

'He certainly seems able to manage to find enough time to interfere with you and Matthew though'.

'Get out,' I snapped. 'I have never heard of anything so outrageous in my entire life. Peter would absolutely never be any of those things that you even dare to say about him'

'All right, I will leave. But be very careful about the amount of time that you let him spend with Matthew alone, until you know more about him than you do now. It takes a very long time before you know someone properly.'

She walked out of the kitchen, slamming the door.

Peter walked in to find me sitting at the kitchen table looking very pale and close to tears.

'What's wrong?'

'It's nothing, really.'

'It doesn't look like nothing.' He sat down beside me and looked at me intently.

'What did your mother say that upset you?' he asked.

I knew instinctively that I couldn't hide anything from him. He seemed to be the kind of person who knew what his instincts told him. I felt very threatened. I would be forced to approach the question of his age, which I was trying to delay for as long as possible.

'My mother gets very possessive if anyone gets involved with me and Matthew,' I said finally. 'She finds it very difficult to trust any men. She seems to think they have some ulterior motive, and even questions their sexuality. Just because she has had bad experiences with relationships she thinks everyone else will be the same. But it has been so hard on our own, without any help. Sometimes it just gets impossible, when he is so lively and I just can't move fast enough to make sure that he doesn't come to any harm. I have been so much happier now I am no longer alone.'

Peter gazed down into my eyes and I found myself staring, dumbstruck into the familiar, kind face.

'I'm here,' he said, gently. 'And I'm not going anywhere.'

I knew that I would have to come clean with him about my age, even if I didn't find out how old he was. His age didn't seem to be an issue although somehow I knew mine was going to be of the utmost importance. I was already becoming aware of inappropriate feelings which I knew were making this issue one which needed to be dealt with before the situation started to get any more out of hand. But I told myself there was no need to find out just yet, it would just have to wait.

We sat together in companionable silence, drinking tea. I didn't want Peter to go away, not ever, but knew it was dangerous to place one's hope in another person. I tried to rationalise the situation. I tried desperately to force myself to stop listening to everything that my emotions told me because my reaction to this devastatingly good-looking youngster was dangerous. I knew that if I didn't get back in control I would put my own well-being, and subsequently that of my son's, in jeopardy. But Peter's gentleness and the warmth in his voice made these fears appear irrelevant, any caution would have to be thrown to the wind. From the way I was feeling, what was happening to me was inevitable and I had no idea of how to deal with it.

'You know I will always be there for you,' Peter tried his best to reassure me. 'You know what the situation's like, and what my job involves. I know you have Matthew, and I realise how hard it is for you, both of you. I know it must be very hard for him. A boy needs to have a man around, and if there is anything that I'm able to do for both of you, then I will.'

But I was starting to feel a lot more awkward, especially since being honest with him about my mother's misgivings.

'I think Matthew and I need to be on our own for a while.'

'Don't worry, everything will be fine. I'm going to be on nights over the next few days, but I will see you soon. If you want me to spend time with Matthew, just let me know and I will be here for both of you, I have to go.'

I had resolved not to tell anybody about the way that I felt, not until the age issue was resolved. But it would be only a matter of time before Peter started to suspect something. In any case I was uncertain of how long I would be able to keep my feelings for him hidden. I just wasn't really sure what those feelings really were. He was very handsome, but that wasn't the most important quality that someone could have. It was the way that he listened to other people, and was capable of being very sympathetic to their needs. He listened to me like I really mattered, like I was attractive and special. I was struggling to tell myself that this was all just part of his medical training, as there was no way that I could allow myself to think that it could possibly ever be anything else.

I felt so vulnerable. I knew that I had made some costly mistakes in the past, and couldn't afford to risk making another. Perhaps Mum had been right, maybe his sexuality was questionable and actually, he knew nothing about why Matthew and I were alone, so how much was I prepared to disclose to him? Would it change the way that Peter felt towards Matthew, or would Peter be so totally disgusted with us, that he'd decide that he couldn't be associated with us any longer?

The thought was intolerable. It was completely unbearable. I knew if I disclosed such information to him, that I'd put our friendship at risk, and could even lose it as well as it being completely inappropriate to have such strong feelings of physical attraction to somebody half my age. My mother was forcing me to confront the age issue, instead of shoving it under the carpet, but I was happier if it stayed there. It was easier to stay in the comfort zone.

I was already finding out that I was resorting to my usual behaviour in relationships, that I pushed people away as soon as they started to get uncomfortably close. So how could I change my perception of this in order to achieve that closeness? Peter would surely understand. Was it likely that he'd be more upset by the fact that I didn't feel able to trust anyone at all, and that he was included in that? Although as an individual, he was probably more trustworthy than anyone I had come across up until then. I just knew that I didn't have enough confidence in myself. I had very little self-esteem, and it wouldn't take very much to totally destroy what little confidence I had left. I wasn't sure enough of how Peter saw me, to even want to put him in the position of hearing the awful truth about my past history. The past is the past. Maybe it was better left there. Presumably Peter had a past, too.

If I tackled my fears that Peter might be a homosexual that would also start to raise issues that I felt much too vulnerable to confront him with. I felt my mother was right in saying that I didn't know him at all and I longed for the chance of some time alone with him. As I always had Matthew with me we hadn't had the chance to talk as adults very much. Maybe it might be an idea to arrange the opportunity to be able to talk to each other on our own. But underneath I still felt as if it would be even better just to let things happen naturally.

I was starting to feel much more awkward round Peter. There were occasions when I started to clam up and just didn't know what to say to him at all. But he somehow knew how to draw me out of myself. Surely it was only a matter of time before he started realising what the real problem was. I thought inviting him over, just to corner him, was definitely a bad idea. As usual I opted for the coward's way out, which was just to let things drift nicely along. If something happens between us I could always approach the issue then. But I still didn't feel very happy with myself for not being honest with him. I remembered my mother's threat: 'If you don't tell him, I will.' But it didn't help my moral dilemma, and I didn't like myself one bit for not doing anything.

There seemed to be a constant knot in my stomach, which changed into feelings of being sick, and this in turn made it more difficult than ever to move around. My emotions were affecting my physical health. The physical symptoms always seemed to get much worse the minute that I started feeling that there was too much stress around for me to handle. As I started collecting my wandering thoughts together the telephone rang, making me jump. My mother was on the other end. This reminded me that I had to do some serious thinking about confronting those things that she seemed to want to challenge me about, although I felt rather reluctant to do so.

Once Matthew was in bed I could have some much needed peace and quiet, and sure enough found that I was a long way from that blissful solitude. Perhaps my mother was right to be cautious about allowing another man to get involved with Matthew, especially without any permanent commitment on his part. My previous relationships always seemed to disintegrate as quickly as they started so my one big fear for Matthew was that he'd grow up thinking that all men ever did to the women in their lives, was to stay for a short time and then just disappear. There had to be a way to protect both of us from getting hurt, and there are some very positive points about having a man with the sort of personality that Peter has around.

I hadn't really given my mother's comments about Peter a second thought. I'd thought that she was only passing a general comment about his attractiveness. It wouldn't have occurred to me that there might be something else, something sinister going on. She knew Daniel's betrayal had cut much deeper than anything else that had ever happened to me.

CHAPTER EIGHT

Peter accepted the invitation to dinner. I wondered whether I should have a candlelit dinner, and really spoil him. On the other hand perhaps not, it might be too obvious. When I was feeling well cooking was one of life's pleasures. It's nice to be giving something to somebody else but how could I make him feel good without it being too obvious? I thought that if you live alone home cooking is always welcome, but Peter was different, he could cook very well which made it harder to decide. He probably thought he should be cooking me a meal.

I was really looking forward to this, almost too much. I had felt so nervous about entertaining before and I was always so excited before seeing Peter. I felt like a small child opening presents on Christmas day, the happiness became overwhelming. I couldn't wait to see him again.

*   *   *   *   *   *   *   *

We were sitting very close together, on the sofa.

'I always appreciate it when anybody takes the trouble to cook for me,' said Peter.

'It was really difficult to know what you might enjoy the most. Most men don't know how to cook, but I know its one of your main hobbies, quite an unusual one.'

'What makes you think it is so unusual, then?' Peter asked.

I hesitated, realising where this might lead.

'Daniel never took the slightest interest in ever eating together as a family, let alone helping. He said it was "Woman's work".'

'Maybe that's true, in some families,' he said. 'But Mum always made a point of including all of us in what she was doing. Take bread making for example. How do you think I learned to do it? It was because she let me watch her while she did it and then let me try for myself. I know Matthew hasn't had the chance of any positive male input like that, and that is one of the main reasons why I wanted to help him, not to mention the fact that my younger brother is his age. Children his age are always such hard work. Mum was always on her own with us.'

'Really?' I was shocked. 'I didn't know.'

'Well, Dad was always working away, travelling. He was in the army, you see, based in India, but they have always lived their separate lives. She might as well have been in your situation.'

'You are the first person I have ever met who feels that men should have an equal amount of responsibility when it comes to domestic duties. Daniel would never lift a finger, and just disappeared off to the pub, even when he could see that I was struggling to give him a nice meal and sort out a screaming baby at the same time.'

The room became deadly quiet. I saw the look of kindness and concern on Peter's face.

'You've had a bad time, haven't you?'

I was so embarrassed by the closeness that I looked away. I couldn't meet his eyes. I didn't want the eye contact. It somehow gave so much of me away to him, that I felt as if I was almost transparent. Even though I was absolutely desperate to be close to Peter there was a part of me that wanted to protect my privacy. The question of the age difference was fast becoming a part of that. But now it had reached the stage of becoming the big secret, on my part at least. I was mindful of my mother's attitude, which had resulted in putting the fear of God in to me. On numerous occasions, I had attempted to bring up the subject naturally, but had become so fearful of the outcome once Peter had discovered the truth about why Matthew and I were alone, that I ended up clamming up completely.

I would still feel sick every time the conversation took a turn towards the subject. I also noticed that the pain in my legs would become much worse. I felt as if there was a giant skeleton in the cupboard – the cupboard of my secret past, to which Peter had the key to unlock the secrets. I wanted to trust somebody for once in my life and I felt I could trust Peter. But the pain that was there at the very thought of what he might end up thinking about us was totally unbearable and the direction in which the conversation turned made me cringe.

'Tell me some more about Daniel. I forgot what you said he did.'

'Daniel didn't do anything,' suddenly aware of how angry this made me feel. 'He was a complete loser. He was a very talented artist - he used to paint wildlife before he had an accident.'

'What accident?' Peter wanted to know.

'Well, a few years ago he became a Hell's angel. He bought himself a motorbike and used to ride it in the country. Anyway, to cut a long story short, a car went into the back of him, he came off and damaged his right leg, and now he is in permanent pain. That was the start of all his problems.' I knew I didn't want this conversation to continue, but it was looking as if I had no choice in the matter, 'Because of his pain, he started drinking too much.' That was all Peter would be able to get out of me for the time being. If he wanted to draw other conclusions as to why Matthew and I were on our own, that was up to him. I wasn't about to volunteer anything more about my past.

'Isn't it funny how different people's temperaments are?' Peter said. Yes, I had noticed.

'Take you and me, for example. No-one could be so different. You are so much more tense than me, and emotional, but maybe that is what I like about you. I am too predictable, and I like some unpredictability – and you are full of surprises. Every time I see you, there is something else to discover.' I became suddenly shy, the idea that he had any thoughts about what I might be like, was inconceivable. The door banged.

'That'll be Mum with Matthew,' I said, rising to go to them.

As I opened the front door, I could tell that my Mum had been upset, just by the tone of her voice, which showed that she was feeling stressed.

'What's the matter?' I asked, as I let them in, and putting a sleeping Matthew in his cot.

'Your son. He's what's the matter. I never thought that I would hear myself say this, Fiona, but I just can't cope with him anymore. He is completely beyond me.'

'It isn't Matthew's fault,' I said angrily.

'Well, you try having him around all the time, screaming and screaming and screaming. I must have tried absolutely everything that I know to get him to stop, and nothing would. These mothers have absolutely no idea of the effects that they have when they leave their child with someone else.'

'It isn't as if you are a complete stranger.'

'That doesn't mean that it's the right thing to do, and a child Matthew's age has no other way of letting the adults know they don't want to be left. The poor little mite was screaming until he was blue in the face.'

'It isn't as though I am out at work all day. I just wanted to talk to Peter on our own, for once.'

'Peter is more important to you than your own son,' said my mother, seething with rage. 'It is obvious that he means everything to you. You are just prepared to drop everything else, just for his sake. I have my rights too, and at my age I am entitled to some peace and quiet. I have already done my bit, and been through everything with you, when you were growing up, never mind having to go through it all over again.'

'For goodness sakes, just calm down, otherwise Peter will hear you.'

'I don't care if he does.'

Sure enough Peter had heard the raised voices, and no doubt he sensed the tension in the atmosphere because he slowly opened the living room door and came out into the hall.

'What's wrong?' he asked me, with his usual concern.

'Nothing.'

'Nothing??!!!' exclaimed my mother, throwing a furious glance at me. 'Nothing? Do you know that I give up all my free time to help Fiona out?'

'I don't think that Fiona has actually got a great deal of choice in the matter,' said Peter trying his best to defend me. 'I was only just thinking that it was a good thing that Matthew has got a granny who could help out; otherwise there is no telling what might happen to him. Fiona, struggling with her pain every single day. I'm sure that most of us haven't got a clue. It's about time we were more sympathetic instead of being ready to condemn disabled people all the time. They have enough to cope with just being disabled, without any of the extra pressure. Fiona needs to know that she can count on you.'

'How DARE you! Of course my daughter knows that she can count on me. I am the one who has been left holding the baby, and picking up the pieces from all her messes. Remember that I don't have anyone to support ME when things are difficult. I've had to learn to stand alone for the last sixteen years. But I have already gone through bringing up my own family, and wasn't expecting to have to start all over again at the beginning.' She turned to me, 'You were not in a position to have Matthew. How could you have been so irresponsible, to have brought a child into the world when you should never have had him? He ought never to have been born.'

I couldn't take any more, and realised that I'd reached breaking point.

'I can't take any more of your criticism. I am sorry that I haven't been the perfect daughter, but at least I tried to keep going, and I have always done my best for Matthew.'

'Shouldn't that be our main priority, here?' said Peter. 'Surely all this shouting is no good for him, or either of you, come to that.' He looked at me, and then turned to my mother.

'Come on, why don't I make you a cup of tea and you can take some deep breaths and calm yourself down?'

'I don't need to be told to "calm down" by somebody who has only just come out of short trousers,' fumed my mother under her breath. However I did notice Peter's words were having some effect, despite herself she was starting to calm down.

Peter signalled me to leave him and my mother on their own.

'Why don't I get us all a cup of tea?' I suggested.

I went and made the drinks, but what I saw when I came back made me drop the tray of hot drinks, smashing all the cups and spilling hot coffee all down me. I dashed upstairs in floods of tears before they could see me. When I had come in the living room Peter and my mother were sitting even closer together than we had been, with their arms around each other, my mother had even put her head on Peter's shoulder.

I couldn't believe my eyes. I told myself to stop being so stupid and irrational. I had had my concerns about being more than half Peter's age and it seemed completely ridiculous that my mother could fall into the same trap. I couldn't take any more. Feelings of complete and utter confusion and jealousy raged inside me. I just wanted to lock myself away from all other human contact and remain alone, forever.

Remaining alone was my only defence mechanism. Never would I get close to anyone – not one single fellow human being. I should never have trusted anyone else. After all, I couldn't trust my own mother. But the biggest mistake that I had made was to have trusted myself. It would seem that I was completely incapable of making a mature judgment and I couldn't judge anybody's character. I obviously didn't have a clue. I would never be able to trust anybody ever again.

I should have read the warning signs. It never occurred to me that my own mother would have an ulterior motive, or Peter for that matter. I suppose I had already made a decision to trust Peter, and my mother had always been there for me. It would never have occurred to me that she was capable of betraying me too.

Human beings are complex creatures when it comes to matters of the heart. Emotions run so high that it becomes difficult to separate them from logic. I think that women are much more emotional than the majority of men seem to be. Men seem to be much more capable of staying in control, and like to think they are maintaining the good old British stiff upper lip, and as for showing someone you really care, well that's just too risky.

One must never show the other person how you really feel, you might get hurt. But I think there is a great deal of truth in saying that you must never trust anyone too much, even the people closest too you. They have the capacity to hurt you too much, more than you'd ever imagine. It was obvious that I was a completely naïve idiot who could be taken for a ride by every opportunist.

CHAPTER NINE

I couldn't sleep at all, not tonight or the night before. I hadn't heard anything from Peter since that evening. I wouldn't blame him if he never wanted to contact me again. Not only that, there was something seriously wrong, something which had never happened before – my instincts told me that it was somehow connected to what was happening to the muscles in my legs.

There was a knock at the door and Mum came in with a cup of tea for me, but when she came in I suddenly found that I couldn't get any words out at all. Somehow the weakness in my face made it impossible to move any part of my mouth and I was absolutely petrified. It must have been because of having been so wound up, I could always tell when my stress level had reached boiling point, my muscles were usually affected in some way or another.

This situation was much more terrifying than anything that had gone before. When I tried to get the words out I couldn't manage more than one syllable. My mother didn't know how to deal with it either. At least she knew that something was wrong; something that was affecting my speech. As it was, I hadn't a clue what to say to her about what I'd seen.

However much I had tried to talk myself into looking at the situation from a sensible point of view I still felt completely vulnerable, mum couldn't fancy Peter herself, surely not? Mum is so concerned about me that she's hardly likely to be interested in Peter in the slightest. Peter is so sympathetic, and has a real gift of being able to empathise with others, he was probably just giving her a shoulder to cry on. There surely could have been no encouragement on his part?

But I couldn't forget how distressed it made me feel. Could I really be so jealous if another woman grabs Peter's attention? To be fair to Peter, I had no claims on his attention. We'd never discussed the possibility of the friendship ever meaning anything else to either of us. In fact he probably hadn't any idea of how intensely I felt whenever he was around. Anyway it doesn't matter now because I won't be hearing from him again. If he hasn't been put off by having to sort my mother out, then he'd definitely been put off by all the things she said about me. He probably thought that we were some completely dysfunctional family. If he's gone now and never comes back then it would jolly well serves me right. Mum accused me of making messes all the time and she was right, it did seem to be the only thing I was good at.

The only thing I could do was let mum get me ready for bed, But I still felt upset. I knew my mother really cared about me. I could rely on her. She'd been there for me through thick and thin; through absolutely everything. It was totally ridiculous – she'd done so much to help me – she'd always been there for me. No matter what, she wouldn't dream of hurting me on purpose. Not ever.

The problem was me. I was over-reacting. That was evident due to the fact that my physical symptoms were deteriorating fast. My emotions had wrecked too many of my relationships with other people. I had to LISTEN and LEARN and LOOK at the bald facts in front of me, not what my raging emotions were telling me as they churned and surged round me in a raging mass. But this time it wasn't just me, my entire family was being affected by them, and I couldn't allow that to happen.

I needed my mother more than ever. But I couldn't handle my own emotions. I certainly didn't want my emotions to entirely destroy my relationship with my mother on a whim. But even these rational, even logical thoughts couldn't stop the pain I was feeling from the sting of Peter's apparent rejection of me. As I tossed and turned I knew that I had to wait to hear from him, and hoped that the post would bring some word from him.

The next morning the letter box rattled, and I knew instantly that the letter waiting to be picked up on the mat would be from him.

Dear Fiona,

I don't know what I've done that's upset you so much. I was upset for both of you. It seems that your mother really cares about you, and only has your best interests at heart, you know. All she wants is the best for you and Matthew.

I did enjoy yesterday. It made a nice change to have some time alone together. Unfortunately, I have to be at work on Monday, but you can phone me on the mobile if you want to talk about anything. (Oh, I forgot that you weren't able to talk, were you?) That's why I'm taking the time to write to you now. I didn't want you to worry about anything that you might have seen on Friday. There was nothing going on as far as I was concerned, I was comforting her, she was in such a state. If I don't hear from you today then I will come round and talk in the next few days. Try not to worry too much, and I hope that you are talking properly again, soon.

Yours,
   Peter.

*   *   *   *   *   *   *   *

After reading Peter's letter it was as if a great burden had rolled away from my shoulders. The episode with my mother made me realise that it wouldn't take much to completely destroy what little confidence I had gained since Daniel's betrayal. The consequences were more devastating than the reality of having to wake up to what my ex-partner was really like.

The emotional turmoil of that night was the worst I have ever experienced. I had feelings towards Peter but I wouldn't allow myself to indulge in them under any circumstances. It was better to pretend they weren't there at all than to risk another chance of being so terribly hurt. I valued my friendship with Peter too highly to put it at risk. But it wasn't just Peter that I couldn't trust;

I also couldn't trust myself any more. That was why I spent so much time trying to analyse what had happened with my mother, I couldn't make any sense out of it. Peter might throw some light on the situation after we'd had the chance to talk about things properly. I thought it called for a long walk down the cycle path, then to the canal where the stillness of the water was so therapeutic and calming that it gave me no alternative but to let go of all the stress and anxiety. Having Peter's gentle personality around as well could only result in a completely relaxing afternoon. So why was I so scared and worried about the prospect of seeing Peter again?

I knew that the friendship had moved beyond the stage of making impressions. I needed to be real with him, if it were to develop into anything remotely meaningful. There was something almost dark and even sinister about the fear lurking in the dark corners of my mind. What was it about Peter that was causing all this anxiety? Was Peter the problem at all? This was troubling me since my relationship with him was one of the most stable experiences in my whole life. It had to come from within me and had nothing to do with him at all. Maybe it came from my knowledge that a relationship with him was out of the question, that his age did matter, and that the excessive range of emotions that I felt whenever he was near me were completely unrealistic.

CHAPTER TEN

The next time Peter had a free afternoon I suggested that it might help to have some fresh air and exercise. As it was a pleasant and sunny day I had prepared a picnic with the thought that we could sit by the canal and watch the narrow boats drifting slowly by.

We walked silently until we reached my favourite place, where there was a huge weeping willow tree, its long green leafy branches hanging over the water's edge. I got out the rug and we sat down in the shadow of the tree. There was very little conversation between us. I sat quietly, watching the ripples of the water as the ducks swam past, followed by two elegant swans with their long necks held high. All my pent up stress and anxiety drained away as I watched them sail past. Words seemed so insignificant. The orange glow from the sunshine turned the water into different shades of oranges and reds, dark, light, and yellow, all mixed up together like a rainbow.

The warm glow from the sun reflected Peter's fairness. Every time I looked at his face I saw something new in his personality. If I were an artist, I thought, watching each facial expression as it was reflected in the light, I would sketch Peter's face, and paint all these shades in different colours. My mind wandered, and I found myself imagining what Peter's fresh white shirt would feel like against my cheek. I just wanted to be able to lay my head on his shoulder, and stay there forever, and ever and ever. Suddenly I was aware of his blue eyes looking intently into my own.

'Fiona, may I ask you something? I know its personal but why do you think your speech came back when I contacted you?'

I didn't know what to say. I wanted to tell him how much I cared for him. That seemed to be the only thing that mattered. But if I said the wrong thing there would be no chance of any happiness now or in the future. Somehow I had to find a way of showing him that I cared, without taking too many risks.

There was no need to reply. Peter's hand was on my shoulder, drawing me towards him. The tension between us was electric. I leant against him, laying my head on his shoulder. We sat together for what seemed to be forever and then it happened. He kissed. Me. It was sweet, and warm, and very, very gentle. There was something so familiar about that kiss, it was like coming home. But I found myself panicking and I broke away, pushing him from me. I was so scared.

'Peter, we mustn't. I can't.'

'Why?' Peter looked hurt. 'I have grown to understand you, I feel protective towards you. What's wrong with showing you that I care?'

'It isn't that.'

It was the age difference. However much I tried to pretend to myself that it didn't matter I couldn't help but wonder what would happen in ten years time when I would be getting on for my mid-fifties? What had happened just now suddenly felt terribly wrong. One of us had to stop the other one from taking things too far. I hadn't before realised that this role could be mine.

'I can't do this Peter. This isn't right. You don't understand.'

'Understand what? If it's about being disabled, then that's the worst reason there is. If I find someone attractive it doesn't make the slightest difference,' Peter said angrily.

'It's nothing to do with that. But my disability is completely unfair on you. I just can't have a relationship and expect you to accept all the limitations that I have to live with, every day. Peter, I couldn't do that to you. I just care for you too much. You deserve something so much better.'

Tears were now flooding down my cheeks.

'Do you really think that matters now,' Peter sounded so concerned. 'Of course it doesn't. I have always been there for you, haven't I? Doesn't that mean something?'

'Yes. I suppose…'

'Well, what's wrong with showing somebody that you care, then?'

'Because the physical side is dangerous,' I said.

But I really wanted to say; 'Because I just wouldn't be able to stop myself, and I have always loved you, right from the beginning'

'One day I will tell you. Let's just stay friends.'

But I knew this wasn't what I really wanted. Not at all. Everything had got to the point of no return. It was the first time I had seen Peter really angry.

'But I know that's not what you really want, Fiona.'

Suddenly he changed into a complete stranger. He became rough and forced me into holding him close. Then pushed me to the ground and lay on top of me. But I was never scared, because underneath I trusted him deeply. This didn't feel wrong. It meant something to both of us. It must do. So I found my body, which had been aching for contact with his for so long, responding.

We melted into each other's bodies as we made love in the warm glow of the sunshine. His warm young arms felt every part of my body. I felt his fresh, young skin against me, as each part of his body touched mine, demanding a response. The sensations he was drawing from me were unlike anything I had ever experienced with Daniel.

After we had finally reached our climax, we just lay in each other's arms, and I knew I loved him. I just loved him so much. But this still didn't feel right, deep down I knew that he could never love me. But for now I could try to kid myself that he did. He didn't, and couldn't, and I had to come out of the denial because that's where I had gone. I had to face the truth: Peter didn't love me, and couldn't ever love me. And neither could anybody else, not ever. I was totally unlovable and unattractive.

CHAPTER ELEVEN

I haven't been able to write for ages. I forget how long it's been since I've been able to use my arms. It's been a month at least, maybe more. I haven't been able to walk around either, and all the time I have been in absolute agony, just sheer, continual agony. The emergency doctor was called out on several occasions and I started having to go to the hospital regularly for tests.

'Don't worry, we will get to the bottom of all this,' the Doctor kept saying.

He was absolutely convinced that I had Multiple-Sclerosis, even more so when my speech kept faltering and so he booked me in for an MRI scan. They showed me round the scanning room which was filled with a big white chute; it reminded me of the tunnel from "Alice in Wonderland".

*　　*　　*　　*　　*　　*　　*　　*

I had a most unfortunate accident the morning of the next scan, which actually landed me in hospital and with an even bigger shock than I had anticipated coping with. I had managed to regain some mobility but my sense of balance had been thrown off course. My coordination had completely gone out of the window, I couldn't feel the floor. Losing my balance I fell, head first from the top of the stairs to the bottom. Then, of course, I couldn't get up at all. There was no movement in either of my legs.

Matthew picked up the phone and dialled my mother's number, but there was no reply. It had been several months since I'd seen her; we hadn't spoken since the incident with Peter. That was my own stupid fault for being so hurt and angry about some of the things that had been said, by both of us, in the heat of the moment that night. And what happened to Peter after that day by the river? He'd gone. I hadn't seen or even heard from him for months. Matthew had no choice but to ring for the ambulance. The paramedics arrived with a wheelchair. Lifting me off the floor, they put blankets round me and put an oxygen mask over my face before wheeling the chair out to the ambulance.

There was a five hour wait in casualty. At half-past five in the morning, the staff eventually decided that I should be admitted onto the ward. I objected because there was really no need, I only had a few scratches and some bruising. But they wouldn't listen. Apparently, I would only have to wait a few more days for results and I needed to stay in hospital all that time to recover. Anyway, the nurses and the doctor came to give me some scan results.

'Well, we've found something,' said the doctor
'Is it negative, again?'
'It's positive.'
'What does that mean?' I thought they had tested me for yet something else.
'You're pregnant!'

I didn't know what to think. I had no idea how I could possibly be. Then I remembered the walk by the water and what had happened afterwards. So that must have been when it had happened. But I hadn't had any contact with Peter for months. I tried his mobile number but got no reply so I left several messages asking him to come and see me urgently. There was still no response. All I could do was wait.

CHAPTER TWELVE

I waited and waited for a phone call. But one didn't come and then one day there was a knock at my front door. Peter was standing outside. I just stared at him. It had been so long since I'd seen him. Seeing him face to face was such a complete surprise, I didn't know what to say to him.

'Aren't you going to invite me in?'

'Did you get my messages?' I asked.

'Yes. But I've been away working for the last few months, in Warwick. Now I'm back here for a month, and then I'm off to America for a year. Anyway, how are you, and how is Matthew?'

'Peter, there is something I need to tell you,' I was petrified of his reaction. 'I've been really ill over the last few months and now they have found something.'

'What have they found?'

'I don't know how to tell you… I'm pregnant.'

Now it was his turn to look shocked.

'How can you possibly be, I haven't seen you for months.'

'As far as I know, it only takes the once,' I said angrily. 'What about what happened before you went away?'

'Oh, that' he said dismissively.

I couldn't believe it. I felt so hurt. All this time I had believed that it meant as much to him as it had done to me, and obviously now, it didn't mean anything at all.

'What are we going to do, Peter?' I asked.

'I would have thought that the most sensible option in your situation would be to have an abortion. You really have no other choice.'

'I can't believe that I'm hearing you say this.' I was now close to tears. 'You are a doctor. I wouldn't have thought that you'd tell anybody to destroy a life.'

'I can't help you.' He'd put on his distant front again.

'Why not? You wanted it too.'

'Yes, ok. I admit it. But things have changed. I'm not going to be in Nottingham for very much longer.'

'So where are you going, then?'

'I told you; to America, for at least a year. I have already signed the contract, and there isn't anything I can do about it now.'

I wanted to be honest with him. I couldn't carry this burden around with me for any longer. Somehow I had to face what was now inevitable. I took deep breaths.

'There is something that I need to tell you. We've got to talk.'

'Well, I've got time. So what is it you want to tell me?'

I looked at him. Whatever happened next, I had nothing to lose. I couldn't bring myself to say anything. But I knew I must. As I forced the words out it felt as if they didn't belong to me. That it was another person that this was happening to. Somehow I was in a dream; that I would suddenly wake up, any minute now.

'I love you, Peter.'

There. That was that. The truth was out in the open. I stopped feeling sick, and the feelings of fear started to drain away. They had been there for months. I waited, terrified, for his response.

'I know,' he said finally. 'I think I always knew.'

He looked at me.

'Fiona, do you think marriage is a viable option?'

'What? Are you asking me to marry you?'

'No. I'm not. I can't ever marry you, I don't love you.'

I felt as if he'd become a total stranger, no longer the warm, caring person I thought I knew. He had a cold, hard sarcastic side to his nature that I'd never seen before.

'Peter, there is something else that I need to tell you about. It's my age. Do you know how old I am?'

'I'd say about thirty-five.'

'No, actually add on about ten years to that.'

All of a sudden I had such a terrible stomach ache that I fell to the ground and just lay there. I thought I was going to pass out. I hadn't fainted, but pains were shooting all over my body. Peter gently helped me off the floor and onto the sofa.

'So that was what I didn't understand.'

'Yes, that you are half my age. But I still love you '

'You've got to forget me,' he said coldly. 'You've just got to.'

'How can I when I can't stop loving you?'

'You'll get over it.'

'It's got harder since you went away, and anyway, what about the baby?'

'I told you before, have an abortion. It's your only option. I'm not going to be around any more. It's fact, I had better go now, and it's fairer on you if I never come back.'

He walked to the front door, opened it, and shut it behind him.

That was the last time I ever saw him.

*   *   *   *   *   *   *   *

I had the abortion. But ever since that moment when I told Peter everything, when I told him the truth, I have walked normally, with no pain. The paralysis has gone completely; I can now lead a normal life. I might have lost the person I loved, but I have regained my physical health, and I can now do things that I could only dream of before.

Dear Peter,

I have missed you so much since you went away, and have not been able to stop thinking about you every single day. Matthew also misses you a lot, and keeps asking when you are coming back. I don't know what to tell him because I sense that you will not return. I know that I have really blown it this time. I knew you were angry with me the last time that we saw you, because there was no connection there - nothing. After everything that we have gone through together, you suddenly seemed so cold, and hard – and distant.

I felt that I was trying to find someone who had once been there but existed no longer – I came away from that meeting and cried solidly for three hours. I knew that something was different, and that it was never going to be the same again.

I have never known you to be so cold towards me, but I knew it must have been because of the baby. I would give everything to make things different. If I could turn the clocks back, I would - I wanted it to be perfect for us.

I love you.
   Fiona

*   *   *   *   *   *   *   *

Dear Fiona,

Thank you for your letter – and my apologies to you for having taken so long to get in touch. As you can appreciate, I had my own reasons for doing this. I know that you are upset, but I don't think that it is a good idea for us to be in continual contact now; as far as I am concerned, things are over between us. You are right to say that you feel that things can never be the same again. There is something that I should have told you, but I didn't want to hurt you. I am getting married to a girl I met at work, she's called Olivia. I hope that you can be happy for me.

I never wanted to cause you any pain, and hope that this will finally help you to put this in the past and that you will be able to move on, as regards your thoughts of me.

Regards,
   Peter

*   *   *   *   *   *   *   *

THE CYCLE PATH

As we travel on life's journey
It takes us down a path
Of rich experiences – that mould us and
Make us into the person that we become at
The end of the journey.

The cycles move forward completing
Life's cycle.
So we reach our goal and hold onto the journey of
Life's rich promises.

THE END

Printed in the United Kingdom
by Lightning Source UK Ltd.
102329UKS00001B/214-312